Legal & Disclaimer

The information contained in this book is not designed to replace or take the place of any form of medication or professional medical advice. The information in this book has been provided for educational and entertainment purposes only.

The information contained in this book has been compiled from sources deemed reliable, and it is accurate to the best of the Author's knowledge. However, the Author cannot guarantee its accuracy and validity so cannot be held liable for any errors or omissions. Changes are periodically made to this book. You must consult your doctor or get professional medical advice before using any of the suggested remedies, techniques, or information in this book.

Upon using the information contained in this book, you agree to hold harmless the Author from and against any damages, costs and expenses, including any legal fees, potentially resulting from the application of any of the information provided by this guide. This disclaimer applies to any damages or injury caused by the use and application, whether directly or indirectly, of any advice or information presented, whether for breach of contract, tort, negligence, personal injury, criminal intent, or under any other cause of action.

You agree to accept all the risks of using the information presented inside this book. You need to consult a professional medical practitioner in order to ensure you are both able & healthy enough to participate in this program.

Contents

Introduction

Nowadays, we do not just want to be lean; we also want strong and healthy bodies. For this reason, we should focus as much on burning fat as on gaining muscle.

Burning fat does not mean we should eliminate it entirely from our diet. What we should do is choose it intelligently and opt for healthy fats, combined with foods that favor digestion. If we want to lose weight healthily, we should burn fat intelligently. This involves eliminating the excesses from our body while also increasing muscle mass.

To achieve this, we will focus on food. Food plays a fundamental role in the distribution of fats in our body. In addition to these tips that will provide in this Book, of course, you must do sports two or three times a week, and combine a cardiovascular routine and strength exercises to tone the muscles. You can achieve this with high-intensity interval exercises, which alternate different types of effort in a few minutes, with a few seconds of rest in between.

In this Book, you will discover 7 Steps to lose fat build muscles. Also, we will provide some recipes that allow you to achieve this goal with the least possible sacrifice and without going hungry.

Enjoy it!!

Chapter 1
Step 1: Foods that activate the metabolism

We all use the word "metabolism." Usually, we have phrases such as "I have lost weight because my metabolism has changed." "I do not lose weight because my metabolism is very slow," or, "you are lucky because you have a very fast metabolism," etc. But, in reality, metabolism is a measurable entity. In simple terms, it is the speed at which you burn calories. It is calculated with a formula and depends on age, sex, height, weight, genetics, lifestyle, hours of sleep, type of work, type of training, the percentage of fat and muscle, the degree of hydration, etc. Come on; it is almost everything!

Among those factors that affect the metabolism are foods that we eat and drink every day. Twofoods with an identical value of calories can produce very different effects on our metabolism. Even foods high in fat and calories can help you burn more calories if you compare their effect on the metabolism with foods low in fat and calories. Below, we'll review the best foods to increase your metabolism and get it to work in your favor when it comes to burning fat and maintaining a strong and toned body.

10 Foods that accelerate the metabolism

Many of us have searched hundreds of times for a list of foods that are rich, healthy and that contribute to losing weight quickly and safely. Well, for this reason, we brought to you these 10 foods that accelerate the metabolism. They are all suitable products that will be very helpful when it comes to improving the correct functioning of your body.

Green apple

Experts say that eating a green apple a day regulates the level of fat in the body. The reason is straightforward. When consuming this fruit, preferably in the afternoon, it will help the metabolism to increase, and thus, calorie burning in the body will increase.

Whitefish

This type of fish is perfect to accelerate the metabolism. Its quick and easy digestion makes it suitable for your body to work a little harder. It is also beneficial, because unlike steak or beef, it's is very soft, and the body can absorb it faster.

Chicken

The chicken, thanks to its large amounts of protein, is conducive to burning calories by increasing the digestive process and thus, body metabolism becomes much faster. Roasted chicken is also an excellent option for consumption as it is low-calorie food.

Green leafy vegetables

Rich in beta-carotene and other nutrients, green leafy vegetables burn that energy you do not need. Broccoli, lettuce, and spinach are recommended for you to eat and include in your diet.

Black coffee

With its active ingredient, caffeine, black coffee is an excellent metabolizer. You must take it without milk and with very little sugar to see the results. This drink is ideal to burn that extra fat that your body does not need.

Egg

It is believed that the egg contains high levels of calories. But it has been proven that egg whites contain no fats but proteins, compounds that are great formaking your body act more effectively when it comes to eliminating fats.

Grapefruit

Grapefruit is rich in vitamins, especially C; it helps eliminate toxins from the body and actively cleanses the liver. It is vital that you consume it so that your body is free of impurities.

Green Tea

Green tea accelerates fat burning and enhances metabolism. Green tea is also ideal to improve your digestion and help with food intake when you eat them.

Spicy Spices

Spicy spices such as chili or red pepper are spectacular to making your metabolism a fast process.

Protein shake

Choose some fruits or food products that contain high protein content; we recommend the almonds, milk, and soy. Make this protein shakes regularly, and you will see excellent results.

It is essential to keep in mind that the increase in metabolism also depends on a balanced diet and an optimal exercise routine. These 10 foods that accelerate the metabolism should be accompanied by an excellent hydration of your body with sufficient amount of water.

Hunger and metabolism

You already know, if you eat little, your metabolism becomes slow, because it adapts to burning fewer calories a day, thus, it is prepared to save reserve fat in times of prolonged hunger. Hunger is the signal that dictates the pace of metabolism, but it is not all that simple, as there is a need for balance. Eating enough nutritious food coupled with good exercise will help hasten your body metabolism. Such a person can easily shed 8000 calories in a 6-hour cycle. The reality is that few people are able toburn such amount of calories in a single day. The same happens if you eat poorly, bad food or junk food, the metabolism does not work because you do not give the body the right nutrients to create muscle mass and prevent fat from accumulating in the reserve areas.

Chapter 2
Step 2: Choose healthy fats

Fats have been demonized for a long time and presented as the main culprit for obesity. Many people, out of ignorance start removing any source of fat entirely from their diets. As one of the essential macronutrients (together with proteins and carbohydrates), today, we know that we need to consume them for the correct functioning of our body: we just have to know how to choose them and determine which the healthiest sources are.

For this reason, in this chapter, you will be able to find sources of healthy fats of different origin, both animal and vegetable, and a few recipes for you to include in your diet.

Healthy fats of plant origin

In the case of fats of vegetable origin, we should avoid the hydrogenated or partially hydrogenated fats. They that are often used in industrial bakery and an example is palm oil.

Instead, we have a wide variety of foods that provide good quality fats:

Avocado: very fashionable lately and one of the most consumed fruits. It is a cool thing to look for avocados that are grown as close as possible to you. It offers you 15 grams of fat per 100 grams of avocado, this being its chief macronutrient. At the time of consuming it, you can do it in the form of the famous guacamole, as an accompaniment to a chicken salad or as a tartar with zucchini and prawns.

Nuts: nuts in all their varieties are the ones that contain more fats in their composition. They contain about 21 grams of fat per 100 grams of nuts. Hazelnuts, pistachios, and almonds are also good choices. To consume them, try making spreadable creams or include them in your salads.

Seeds: both sunflower seeds and pumpkin or sesame seeds contain a good amount of healthy fats, and you can use them as toppings in your breakfast smoothies bowls. Also, chia seeds, very fashionable lately, can help you increase the number of healthy fats in your diet.

Olives: and, obviously, the olive oil that comes from them. Olives contain Omega-3 and Omega-6 essential oils, as well as a good amount of vitamins A and C. You can consume them in different ways, for example preparing spreads such as tapenade, in the form of an appetizer or including them in your salads (of chickpeas, olives, tomato, and cheese). When it comes to consuming olive oil, it is best to opt for extra virgin, since it contains a greater amount of Omega-3 and Omega 6, in addition to more vitamins E.

Legumes such as soybeans and peanuts: You cannot leave legumes aside when talking about healthy fats. Soy is the legume that contains more healthy fats (more than 18 grams of fat per 100 grams of this legume), while peanuts contain lesser amount at 14 grams of fat per 100 grams of food. As ideas to consume them, we propose a tasty salad of spinach and chicken with soy; scrambled tacos of spicy tofu; or prawns with curried peanut butter.

Healthy fats of animal origin

Bluefish: The healthiest option when looking for fats of animal origin is found in blue or naturally fatty fish, which contain a large amount of Omega-3. This unsaturated acid helps you prevent heart disease by protecting your heart.

It is present in fish such as salmon, sardines, bonito, tuna or swordfish; which you can prepare in the following ways:

- Terrine of salmon and dill cheese

- Tuna in curry mango sauce

- Pickled sardines

- Norwegian salmon glazed with sake and teriyaki

- Light tuna quiche

- Smoked sardines with tomato and its gelatin

- Prepared with oil, lemon, and rosemary

- Farfalle salad with swordfish, olives, and capers

Eggs: about 70% of the egg's calories come from the fats it contains, but it is monounsaturated fats (approximately 8.5 grams of fat in each egg). Also, it provides other essential micronutrients such as phosphorus, potassium or vitamin A. If you are looking for new ideas to consume it, do not miss the ideas that we give you in this chapter.

Chapter 3
Step 3: Improve the assimilation of fats

Usually, when we eat, we only think about how good the food is or how hungry we are. We never stop to think about the way in which food travels through our digestive system or the way it decomposes into molecules that our body uses in various processes.

The truth is that eating is more than putting food in your mouth. And what you do besides eating food can affect the way your body absorbs nutrients.

Fortunately, there are ways to help the body improve its ability to absorb nutrients, and thus, you make better use of food and improve the functions of your body.

Why are nutrients important?

Nutrients are needed to generate critical biochemical reactions in the body that are vital to our health and well-being. And your bodies work thanks to a combination of micronutrients, macronutrients and the water you consume.

Thisis achieved with protein, carbohydrates, fats, vitamins, minerals and, of course, water. If you have a balanced and complete diet, you nourish your body; you give calcium to your bones to keep them strong. Your muscles grow thanks to your protein intake, and your organs function thanks to the vitamins and minerals that come from fruits and vegetables.

If you do not eat a large variety of nutrients, you run the risk of missing some nutrients, which would affect the biochemical reactions of your body. You need nutrients so that all of your organs function healthily: the heart, the brain, the liver, the kidneys, and the thyroid, just to name a few.

The symptoms of nutritional deficiency can be very subtle, such as fatigue, dull hair, or skin blemishes; it can take years for them to become a serious disease.

How does the body absorb nutrients?

For the nutrients to be absorbed, the food has to go through a chemical and mechanical digestion process. After the food passes through your mouth, the digestive enzymes help to break down the molecules of the food.

This breaks down the macro and micronutrients. For example, proteins breaks down into several amino acids, and the carbohydrates are transformed into glucose that is used as energy that is used or stored in reserve.

Once food becomes vital nutrients, it travels to the small intestine and is absorbed by the circulatory system, so the circulatory system is responsible for transporting the nutrients to the different parts of the body that need them.

For this absorption process to work optimally, you need a healthy digestive system. If your digestion or the health of your stomach is not right, then you cannot absorb the nutrients well. Some factors like chewing food well, a reasonable level of hydrochloric acid, stomach bacteria, and a decent cellular integration of the stomach are necessary for the absorption of nutrients.

What factors can negatively affect the absorption of nutrients?

Many factors can negatively affect the digestion in the stomach and the absorption of nutrients from food. These include gastrointestinal problems such as irritable bowel syndrome and celiac disease, as well as a diet high in sugars and processed foods.

Processed foods are low in nutrients, and high in sugars that can steal nutrients from the body, especially magnesium. Some medications such as antacids; medications to control blood pressure; antidepressants and hormones can interfere with the level of nutrients in the body.

Stress and alcohol consumption can affect digestion and absorption of nutrients. Stress increases our nutrient needs, particularly vitamin C, B vitamins and magnesium, which can cause irritability and fatigue if these nutrients are lacking.

Alcohol consumption is related to the reduction of digestive enzymes, so people who drink a lot can limit the breakdown of nutrients in food.

If there are changes in your stool, digestion or energy levels, and in the appearance of your hair, skin, and nails, check with your doctor to see if you have no nutritional deficiencies.

How to improve the absorption of nutrients?

If you do not have any health problems as explained above, there are some ways to improve the absorption of nutrients.

1. Include a variety of foods at each meal

To ensure a combination of nutrients, try to include foods of "many colors" in your diet. For example, salad with roasted vegetables or fried brown rice with carrots, lettuce, pepper, squash, and celery.

Eat different types of food every day and avoid eating the same food, for example, eat different things every day, stir foods, and make sure you include a variety of nutrients.

2. Combine foods rich in vitamin C with iron

People who get iron from plant-based foods (legumes, tofu, dried fruit) can combine them with foods rich in vitamin C to help convert non-heme iron to a form that can be better absorbed.

Eat foods rich in vitamin C such as oranges, peppers, chili, cauliflower and Brussels sprouts along with iron-rich foods (such as legumes and red meat) to increase iron absorption.

3. Include healthy fats in each food

Healthy fats are needed to be able to absorb vitamins such as A, D, E, and K because they are fat-soluble.

As such, you can use dressings with linseed oil or olive oil to improve the absorption of the fat-soluble vitamins in your vegetables. Nuts, seeds, and avocados in salads and meals are excellent for increasing nutrient absorption.

4. Take a probiotic

Nourish your gut, especially if you have digestive problems like irritable bowel or constipation, it's the best thing you can do for a start. You can do this if you fill your intestine with healthy bacteria through probiotics or foods rich in probiotics.

5. Avoid drinking tea at lunchtime

Although tea contains polyphenols and other compounds that may help reduce the risk of chronic diseases, these compounds also inhibit iron absorption. Avoid taking tea and coffee with food because they can inhibit the absorption of many vitamins and minerals.

6. Reduce caffeine and alcohol

Alcohol and diuretics (like coffee) not only limit the number of digestive enzymes in our system, they also damage the linings of the stomach and intestinal cells, and make it more difficult for nutrients to pass from the digestive system to the bloodstream.

Better still, try to incorporate fruits and vegetables that have natural digestive enzymes like pineapple, papaya, and some mushrooms.

7. Control your stress levels

Believe it or not, stress negatively affects digestion. The cortisol in the body during stress states causes digestion to be slower, and the food remains undigested in the system.

To help, try taking deep diaphragm breaths that relieve stress and make the digestive system work.

8. Hydrate

This one crucial factor can aid or stop digestion. When you do not have enough fluids or water, you notice the difference in your stool; your digestive system depends on the level of hydration because the blood cannot transport the nutrients if it does not have enough water.

Natural remedies to better digest fats

Below you can learn some basic tips to better assimilate the bad fats you consume and thus facilitate the digestive process of your body. This can translate to more favorable conditions for those who want to lose weight. In any case, it is better not to take a diet that contains bad fats.

1. Apple cider vinegar

Apple cider vinegar is a powerful fat burner that is regularly used in household cleaning precisely because of this characteristic. Apple cider vinegar is an essential food if you are looking for a high-quality natural product so that the digestion of fats is optimal.

2. Green tea and red tea

Green tea or red tea, are two types of infusions that you can drink every day. They are even more important if you want to lose weight by assimilating fats better, once you have finished eating. In case you suffer from anemia, you will have to separate them from your food since sometimes they prevent the iron from assimilating. But without a doubt, these two liquids are highly recommended for faster digestion of fats.

3. Lemon juice

Lemon juice is one of the main ingredients to consider if you would like to treat the fats that the body receives. It helps to neutralizestomach acids, and therefore, you will digest fats better, and you can also improve the pH of the body.

4. Artichoke extract

To cap it up, we want to provide ideal working conditions for the liver,and for this, the artichoke will help you. Whether cooked, baked or infused, the properties of the artichoke will benefit the liver and are also a great help to lose weight. If you opt for the infusion, it is advisable to mix with some water and take it with meals.

Chapter 4
Step 4: Good quality protein

Our body needs a certain amount of quality proteins daily for basic functions such as growth or the formation and regeneration of cells.

On the one hand, there are foods such as fish, eggs, and dairy which provide much more protein than any other nutrient, in addition to presenting a high nutritional value. These are classified as good quality proteins or also as clean proteins. On the other hand, there are foods such as cereals, pulses (except soy) and nuts that do not reach the quality or biological value of the previous ones.

What makes a protein of good quality?

The quality of a protein depends on the combination of amino acids and their digestibility. Digestibility is a way of measuring the use of food, that is, the ease with which it is converted in the digestive system into substances useful for nutrition. Amino acids are very small particles that bind together to form proteins. They can bind from 2 to hundreds of amino acids, and this is what determines the formation of small enzymes or even complex tissues and organs.

The type of amino acids that make up a protein is what determine its functions. Everybodys' genetic code contains a combination of amino acids that make up our entire body. For instance, in hair cells, there is a combination of amino acids that people must have to make curly or straight hair, as the case may be.

This is how accurately this informationis stored in all our cells and how vital the presence of amino acids in our body. Although, our body manufactures some of them known as "non-essential" amino acids, but there are others that we cannot manufacture. Hence, we have to obtain them from the diet. These are the so-called "essential" amino acids (isoleucine, leucine, lysine, methionine, phenylalanine, threonine, tryptophan, valine, histidine and arginine).

For a protein to be of good quality, it must provide all the essential amino acids, because if it lacks one, it becomes a protein of poor quality. Vegetable proteins such as legumes (beans, lentils, chickpeas, etc.) and cereals (rice, corn, wheat, etc.) are considered to be of poor quality. Some of them have the essential amino acids that are missing in others. But then, they complement each other perfectly, and must be consumed together to raise their nutritional quality.

On the other hand, animal proteins are of good quality because they provide all the essential amino acids. However, there are on different levels, which is dependent on their level of digestibility, as this will depend on the correct absorption of their amino acids and nutrients in general. Animal proteins have the highest nutritional value because it has the most balanced proportions of the ten essential amino acids whose digestibility is very good. A typical example is cow milk.

Cow milk is made up of two types of proteins: casein, and whey.

Milk casein has a very important nutritional role since in addition to providing essential amino acids; it is the one that contributes the highest amount of calcium and phosphorus to the diet. These minerals are essential for the formation of bones and the correct storage of energy in all our cells.

Whey proteins, on the other hand, are mainly albumins and globulins. They provide a type of amino acids that are difficult to find in other sources of protein, the famous branched chain amino acids which:

- they make up 35% of our muscle mass

- help to constantly synthesize new muscle fibers

- help to recover and maintain healthy muscles after exercise.

A deficient consumption of this type of amino acids results in malnutrition and loss of muscle mass. From the age of 40, we started to lose muscle mass gradually (0.5 - 1% per year), which translates into a loss of almost 50% at 80 years, bringing with it serious consequences such as bone fragility, weakness, and fatigue.

Consumption of proteins like those that are present in milk (lactalbumins), has shown that it can help reduce the rate of muscle loss and we must include them daily in our diet because thanks to them we develop, grow and manage to maintain good physical health and mental wellbeing. So when you plan your meals, include this type of food so that you and your family stay well nourished.

Top 5 Foods with high-quality proteins to gain muscle

Choosing good protein sources when you want to improve your physical appearance is one of the main keys to achieving good results.

There are 3 types of macronutrients: fats, proteins, and carbohydrates. Proteins are formed by amino acids, which are the "blocks" of this, if you want to gain muscle mass or prevent its loss when you lose weight, you must provide a good amount of amino acids to your body. The supply of amino acids puts your body in a kind of anabolic state, or rather, helps to maintain a positive nitrogen balance.

In addition, amino acids such as leucine, are very good for increasing blood insulin levels, which helps to provide nutrients to the muscle cell and reduce protein catabolism or loss of lean mass.

There are 2 types of amino acids, the essential ones which the body needs to be provided through food and the non-essentials, which can be manufactured by your body from other amino acids.

The non-essential amino acids are glutamic acid, arginine, serine, alanine, tyrosine, cysteine, glycine, asparagine, proline, aspartic acid, glutamine and cysteine and the essential amino acids are histidine, isoleucine, valine, leucine, tryptophan, lysine, methionine, phenylalanine, threonine and alanine.

The primary amino acids that intervene in the gain of muscle mass are leucine, isoleucine, and valine.

Depending on the number of essential amino acids that a food has, it will determine its biological value. The higher it is; the better it is for your diet. There are 4foods with proteins with a high biological value.

1) The eggs

The biological value is a number that goes from 1 to 100, and the eggs along with the yolk, have a biological value of 100. This food is especially rich in leucine; we also have that egg whites which has a biological value of 88. They are very cheap food and available to everyone. It should be noted that if they are not heated, the peptide bonds formed between the amino acids are not broken, so in this case, the absorption of protein would be greatly reduced, up to 50%.

2) Whey

Whey is what powdered proteins are madeof. This serum is a by-product of the manufacture of cheese and other dairy products. Its biological value is also 100, that is, all its protein is efficiently absorbed. This type of protein is the richest in BCAA, branched chain amino acids, which are isoleucine, valine, and leucine, the most important to gain muscle mass.

3) Beef

Beef is very good because even though it has a biological value of 69, it is rich in arachidonic acid, which helps in the gain of muscle mass. It increases the amount of PG2 and therefore the activity of the satellite cells. If this activityis increased, more muscle is gained since they are more linked to free androgens in the blood.

4) Chicken and turkey

The food of the bodybuilder with a biological value of 79, the turkey is very rich in tryptophan, which is good to maintain a good mood, sleep, etc. They are also foods that are digested very easily and allow a great combination of recipes, and they are quite cheap.

What about foods with vegetable proteins?

Vegetable proteins are not good for gaining muscle because they lack some essential amino acid for our body. In case of being vegan, combining rice and legumes and nuts with soy milk to obtain complete proteins, in addition to using a supplement of vegetable protein powder, such as pea or brown rice protein, phytoestrogens of soy milk usually cause a decrease in DHT, giving us a more gain of fat and fluids.

Chapter 5
Step 5: Reduce carbohydrates

When it comes to reducing carbohydrate consumption, we must bear in mind that the worst are the simple ones, while the complex ones are satiating and have a greater nutritional contribution.

Low-carbohydrate diets were an option that was booming a few years ago. These dietsseek to reduce the consumption of foods rich in carbohydrates and with a lower glycemic index, i.e., those with less impact on sugar levels in the blood. Many people really feel positive changes in their physical well-being by following this diet.

But controlling the level of carbohydrates you consume can be difficult, since many things that you are used to eating are full of these carbohydrates, such as bread, pasta, and so on.

Daily consumption of carbohydrate sources is essentialfor people who want to maintain a healthy body.

It is important to include it in a diet plan in order to enjoy optimal physical and mental performance and maintaina good functioning of the metabolism. However, when it comes to losing body fat, it is necessary to limit the consumption and opt for those foods that contain them in minimal amounts.

Although it is not convenient to suppress them, however, it is of vital importance to learn how to choose the healthiest, that is, the complex ones. Also, it is convenient to implement some tips and tricks which, without endangering our health, can help safely reduce carb intake.

In this chapter, we will show you several of them so that you begin to take them into account each day.

Tips for reducing carbohydrates

1-Tthe consumption of sugary drinks is your worst enemy

Juices and sugary soft drinks that they distribute in the market do not offer a significant nutritional value and, instead, they contribute a large number of calories which are not necessary.

When ingested, an anxiety reaction is generated in the body that, almost always provokes the need for simple carbohydrates. To worsen things, its high sugar content affects metabolic functioning and:

- Increase in insulin resistance.

- Developing type 2 diabetes.

- Increases weight and obesity.

2-Increase the consumption of vegetables

By increasing the daily intake of vegetables without starch, you can reduce the need forconsumption of more carbohydrates that are harmful to the body. Veggies help in improving digestion, increase metabolism and slow food cravings.

Try to choose varieties such as:

- Green leafy vegetables

- Tomatoes

- Carrots

- Beet

3-Increase the intake of healthy fats

Increasing the consumption of foods which have high healthy fats is a decent way to reduce the number of carbohydrates without affecting the energy levels of the body. This type of nutrient is vital for a good metabolic functioning and, in turn, influences the increase in the sensation of satiety.

Some of its best sources are:

- Extra virgin olive oil

- Natural avocados

- Nuts products

- Fatty fish

- Seeds

4-Ensures adequate protein consumption

Although many things have been said about proteins; it is recognized that they are fundamental to enjoy good health and body weight. Your daily consumption of foods containing this nutrient should correspond to 35% calories, and you should include them in breakfast.

Since they are of high energetic value, they will help to have a better performance and, at the same time, they will support the metabolic activities. Below are a few protein source:

- Eggs

- Lean meats

- Fatty fish

- Nuts

- Whole grains

- Legumes

5-Opt for whole foods

Their high fiber content and capacity to absorb water increase the sensation of satiety and facilitate the follow-up of hypocaloric or slimming diets. Whole foods are a good resource for weight loss. This is not because they provide less energy, but because they swell with fluids and produce the impression of filling before continuing to take more food and more calories.

In addition, this variety of foods contains fiber, antioxidants, and other essential nutrients that contribute to improving physical and mental well-being.

6-Substitute the cow milk

Cow milk is an excellent food at a nutritional level due to its large amount of vitamins such as A, D, B1, B2,and its high mineral content. But it has a high content of fat and carbohydrate which makes it bad for weight loss.

Each glass of cow milk gives the body between 12 and 13 grams of carbohydrates, in addition to a significant number of calories. Therefore, it is convenient to replace it with vegetable milk which, unlike this one, only contain little amount of carbohydrates.

There are a lot of varieties that you can choose such as:

- Coco

- Almonds

- Rice

- Nuts

It is important to design and control calorie consumption since this help to combat excess weight. Make sure you include all the nutrient groups in your diet.

Chapter 6
Step 6: Good posture

Good posture is the result of proper body alignment of the spine, muscles, joints, ligaments and other body bones. This organized placement of the different parts of the human anatomy allows the body to use the minimum of effort to perform a physical activity, both in motion and in a static position.

When you have good posture, your body can function in a more efficient way when doing any physical activity, be it running, dance, exercising, standing or sitting. A healthy posture allows you to perform that physical activity more effectively.

Good posture is essential for health because:

- Keeps bones and joints in proper alignment so that muscles can perform their function properly.

- Gives the necessary strength to do any physical activity without putting unnecessary stress on any part of the body.

- Prevents fatigue because the muscles function more efficient, using the minimum of effort.

- Helps to have a more flexible body.

- Keeps the body free of injuries.

- Prevents back pain, neck and shoulder pain, and; muscle aches.

- Avoid abnormalities in the spine, which later could cause serious health problems.

- Reduces the deterioration of the surface of the joints, a symptom that could cause arthritis.

Guide to maintain a correct posture

You must not maintain proper posture when you exercise, but you must be aware of your own body at any time and place. Waiting or standing in the supermarket queue, or sitting down while the subway is coming are also occasions in which you must take care of your posture.

We will give you the key points to keep in mind to maintain good posture while standing, sitting, walking, running and sleeping. Let's review the most important data:

If you are sitting: back straight, shoulders back and down, and soles of the feet resting on the ground. Remember that crossing the legs can hinder circulation and make you suffer from swollen or tired legs.

If you are standing: chest up and abdomen activated since the abdominal muscles are those that help you to stabilize. Knees a little flexed, and body weight distributed between the two legs.

When walking: keep the head up and the neck erect, and avoid looking at the floor, as it can cause cervical pain. Make sure you step on the ground correctly: first with the heel of the foot, then move towards the tip.

When running: the elbows should be bent at right angles so that the movement of the arms accompanies the movement of the legs. You must land with the middle part of the foot (never receive the impact with the heel) and move towards the digits to spread the impact of the shock.

When sleeping: a correct position to sleep is on the side and with the legs shrunk since it is what keeps your spine aligned correctly. Sleeping on a good mattress, and changing it when necessary, is vital to getting a quality rest.

How can you improve your position?

To maintain a correct posture, it is vital that you are aware of your body at all times: realizing that you are misaligned without needing to feel pain is the first step towards a correct posture and a higher quality of life.

Certain disciplines such as Pilates help you to become aware of each part of your own body, make them function independently and globally. Body alignment is one of the basic principles of the Pilates method that should be practiced in each session.

But also in other sports, you must take care of your body alignment: if you work with free weights, you should not start a movement, especially if you use heavy loads until you are well aligned. In activities such as spinning, in which you maintain the same position over a longperiod of time, it is important to receive the appropriate indications on the correct posture.

The toning of the muscles is also very important when maintaining a good posture: strong muscles, dense bones and joints with a good range of movement will make you more effective and efficient in your day-to-day movements.

Body alignment in good posture

Body alignment in good posture requires that all parts of the body be in balance. This means that the weight of the body is well distributed among all the parts.

The alignment in a good posture changes according to what the body is doing but always follows the same principles. In a neutral standing position, these are the main characteristics of a correct alignment:

Feet: Feet are the lower base of your posture. In a neutral standing position, the feet should follow the same imaginary vertical lines that follow the hips and shoulders. They should look forward. The weight of the body should be distributed equally in both feet and in all parts of the sole of each foot.

Knees: The knees should be slightly bent, not too extended or too bent. The knees should face forward, following the same imaginary vertical line that passes through the center of the feet.

Pelvis: The pelvis is the base of your posture. It must be centered with the rest of the body, neither too far forward nor too far back. In proper alignment, the pelvis maintains the natural curvature of the spine. The curvature in this region is inward of the column.

Hips: The hips should follow the same imaginary vertical lines that follow the shoulders and feet.

Trunk: The trunk should be in balance with the pelvis, without being too far forward or too far back. In proper alignment, the pelvis maintains the natural curvature of the spine. The curvature of this region is out of the body.

Shoulders: The shoulders should be relaxed backward. The shoulders follow the same imaginary vertical lines that follow the feet and hips.

Arms: The arms hang relaxed on each side of the body, but they are not flaccid. The arm muscles are active in this position without unnecessary tension.

Head: The head should be erect with the chin in a line parallel to the ground. It must be centered with the imaginary horizontal line that the shoulders follow. The ears should follow the same imaginary vertical line that the shoulders follow.

The muscles in the posture

Muscles are also important in good posture. They are essential to maintaining proper body alignment. The muscles support the spine, pelvis and other organs.

The key with muscles, when it comes to good posture, is that they have enough strength and flexibility to support the bones and organs. The level of strength and flexibility of the muscles should be equal on the left and right side of the body, and on the ventral and dorsal plane of the body.

When the muscles are weaker on one side than on the other, the body cannot maintain proper alignment and goes out of balance. If not corrected in time, this type of muscle imbalance can cause serious postural problems.

Chapter 7
Step 7: Beware of injuries

Exercise is good for you, but sometimes you can hurt yourself when you play sports or exercise. Accidents, wrong exercises or the use of inappropriate clothing and equipment can be some of the causes. Some people get hurt because they are not in shape. Failure to warm up or stretch the muscles can also cause injuries.

The most common sports injuries are:

- Strains and strains

- Knee injuries

- Muscle inflammation

- Achilles tendon injuries

- Pain in the bone of the tibia

- Shoulder rotator cuff injuries

- Fractures

- Dislocations

So, if you get hurt, stop practicing sports or exercise. Continuing to play or keep exercising can cause more damage. The treatment usually begins with the RICE method (Rest, Ice, Compression, andElevation). It helps to relieve pain, reduce inflammation and accelerate healing. Other possible treatments include painkillers, immobilizing the injured area, rehabilitation and, sometimes, surgery.

Follow these steps to avoid possible sports injuries and to continue doing sports:

1. Wear protective equipment, such as a helmet, gloves, knee pads and the like.

2. Warm up before playing sports.

3. Know and respect the rules of the game.

4. Keep others in mind.

5.   Stop playing sports when you get injured.

Wear protective gear

For protective equipment, you must identify what you can wear that can help you avoid hurting yourself. The specific equipment you should wear will depend on the type of sport you practice. The helmet is the most used protective element. It protects your head, a very important part of your body. You must use a helmet when you play rugby, jockey or baseball or when you ride a bike, skate or go skateboarding, to mention a few sports!

Make sure you wear the right helmet for the sport you practice. For example, do not ever wear a baseball helmet to play rugby! They should fit well but without squeezing and, if you are wearing a leash, like in cyclists' helmets, you should tie it. Failure to do this will cause the helmet to fall off at some point during the activity.

Other sports require eye protectors, mouth guards, knee pads, wrist guards and elbow pads, as well as protectors of the inguinal area (only for boys). And do not forget your feet. To play rugby, baseball and soccer you need a special footwear that has rubber or plastic studs on the sole that allow you to grip the ground better when running.

Talk to your parents or your coach to find out what equipment you need. And always wear it when you play sports.

Warm up before playing sports

It is not a good idea to throw yourself into the field and start playing just like that. You should not even start stretching without having warmed up before. So do a little jogging to loosen up your muscles and get ready to play sports.

Know and respect the rules of the game

The traffic lights at the intersections help prevent crashes between the many cars and trucks that circulate on the streets at the same time. Traffic lights are useful because drivers know traffic rules and respect them - at least, most of the time. The same thing happens with sports.

When players know and respect the rules of the game - what is and what is not allowed to; there are fewer injuries. If you know the rules of the game, both you and the other players will know what you can expect from each other. For example, in football, you cannot attack from behind, jump to the legs of a player or touch the ball with your hands. It is allowed - and it is safer - to run after the ball, instead of behind the players.

In sports where plays are used, it helps to understand what each play consists of, and the role each player. Understanding your roles in a play can help you not only to properly enjoy the game but to stay out of harm. Being where you are supposed to be can also help you avoid potential injuries.

Keep others in mind

Some rules of the game have nothing to do with scoring points or committing fouls. Some rules are about how to protect others, respect them and be educated with them. For example, in baseball, the batter cannot throw the bat after hitting the ball and running to first base. You must drop it so that it cannot hurt someone. In the same way, a swimmer should make sure that there is no one in the pool where they want to dive. Otherwise, it could fall on top of another swimmer.

One way to keep others in mind is to communicate in the field. For example, a baseball player in the yard may shout "mine" to avoid a collision with another gardener. Following your coach's instructions during the game can also help you avoid possible injuries. It is also good to be educated, for example, by telling someone that he is wearing the shoelaces untied. Also, check that your laces are securely tied!

Stop playing sports when you get injured

This rule is really important. If you love playing sports, it may seem tempting to keep playing after an injury. But playing sports immediately after injuring yourself or before you've fully recovered from a previous injury is a bad idea. It could aggravate the injury, which would force you to stay without playing sports for a long time. If you injure yourself doing sports, inform your parents and your coach. If necessary, go to the doctor and follow his instructions on when and how you can return to sports.

Now you know what you have to do to avoid injury when they play sports. With a bit of luck, if you follow rules 1, 2, 3 and 4, you will not need to follow the fifth. Or, at least, not very often!

Conclusion

In many occasions, the society's perception on the optimal way to lose fat does not usually align with the dictates of science, something that is mainly due to the false myths about how to lose weight to the advertising stratagems of the industry of fitness and nutrition.

To burn fat and lose weight, it is not necessary to erase them from your diet since they are an essential part of your dietary needs and fundamental to maintaining a healthy hormonal balance. Avoid trans-fats, industrial foods, and added sugars, but opt for healthy sources of fat such as avocados, olives, and bluefish such as salmon or nuts.

Losing fat from a specific body area is physiologically impossible. When we lose fat, we do it integrally.

Remember that the fact you focus on doing a more intense muscular work in a specific area will not make you lose more fat in that area. So, forget about the idea that doing a thousand abdominals a day will give you a toned abdomen. You cannot abandon or ignore the importance of having healthy nutritional habits.

Therefore, we recommend that you opt for multiarticular exercises and that you do not focus exclusively on aerobic work to lose weight and gain muscle. Also, include strength exercises in your weekly training routine.

Philip Cooper

9 781984 980380